How to Live 100 Years

or, Discourses on the Sober Life

How to Live 100 Years
or, Discourses on the Sober Life

Being the Personal Narrative of

Luigi Cornaro

(1464-1566 A.D.)

WORLD LIBRARY CLASSICS

HOW TO LIVE 100 YEARS

Published in 2009 by WLC Books.

The First Discourse

On a Temperate and Healthful Life

It is universally agreed, that custom, in time, becomes a second nature, forcing men to use that, whether good or bad, to which they have been habituated; in fact, we see habit, in many instances, gain the ascendancy over reason. This is so undeniably true, that virtuous men, by keeping company with wicked, often fall into the same vicious course of life. Seeing and considering all this, I have decided to write on the vice of intemperance in eating and drinking.

Now, though all are agreed that intemperance is the parent of gluttony, and sober living the offspring of abstemiousness; yet, owing to the power of custom, the former is considered a virtue, and the latter as mean and avaricious; and so many men are blinded and besotted to such a degree, that they come to the age of forty or fifty, burdened with strange and painful infirmities, which render them decrepit and useless; whereas, had they lived temperately and soberly, they would in all probability have been sound and hearty, to the age of eighty and upward. To remedy this state of things, it is requisite that men should live up to the simplicity dictated by nature, which teaches us to be content with little, and accustom ourselves to eat no more than is absolutely necessary to support life, remembering that all excess causes disease and leads to death. How many friends of mine, men of the finest understanding and most amiable disposition, have I seen carried off in the flower of their manhood by reason of excess and overfeeding, who, had they been temperate, would now be living, and ornaments to society, and whose company I should enjoy with as much pleasure as I am now deprived of it with concern.

In order, therefore, to put a stop to so great an evil, I have resolved, in this short discourse, to demonstrate that intemperance is an abuse which may be removed, and that the good old sober living may be substituted in its stead; and this I undertake the more readily, as many young men of the best understanding have urged upon me its necessity because of many of their parents having died in middle life, while I remain so sound and hearty at the age of eighty-one. These young men express a desire to reach the same term, nature not forbidding us to wish for longevity; and old age, being, in fact, that time of life in which prudence can be best exercised, and the fruits of all the other virtues enjoyed with the least opposition, the senses then being so subdued, that man gives himself up entirely to reason. They besought me to let them know the method pursued by me to attain it; and then finding them intent on so laudable a pursuit, I resolved to treat of that method, in order to be of service, not only to them, but to all those who may be willing to peruse this discourse.

I shall therefore give my reasons for renouncing intemperance and betaking myself to a sober course of life, and declare freely the method pursued by me for that purpose, and then show the good effect upon me; from whence it will be seen how easy it is to remove the abuse of free living. I shall conclude, by showing the many conveniences and blessings of temperate life.

I say, then, that the heavy train of infirmities which had made great inroads on my constitution were my motives for renouncing intemperance, in the matter of too freely eating and drinking, to which I had been addicted, so that, in consequence of it, my stomach became disordered, and I suffered much pain from colic and gout, attended by that which was still worse, an almost continual slow fever, a stomach generally out of order, and a perpetual thirst. From these disorders, the best delivery I had to hope was death.

Finding myself, therefore, between my thirty-fifth and fortieth year in such unhappy circumstances, and having tried everything that could be thought of to relieve me, but to no purpose, the physicians gave me to understand that there was one method left to get the better of my complaints, provided I would resolve to use it, and patiently persevere. This was to live a strictly sober and regular life, which would be of the greatest efficacy; and that of this I might convince myself, since, by my disorders I was become infirm, though not reduced so low but that a regular life might still recover me. They further added, that, if I did not at once adopt this method of strict living, I should in a few months receive no benefit from it, and that in a few more I must resign myself to death.

These arguments made such an impression on me, that, mortified as I was, besides, by the thought of dying in the prime of life, though at the same time perpetually tormented by various diseases, I immediately resolved, in order to avoid at once both disease and death, to betake myself to a regular course of life. Having upon this inquired of them what rules I should follow, they told me that I must only use food, solid or liquid, such as is generally prescribed to sick persons; and both sparingly. These directions, to say the truth, they had before given me, but I had been impatient of such restraint, and had eaten and drank freely of those things I had desired. But, when I had once resolved to live soberly, and according to the dictates of reason, feeling it was my duty as a man so to do, I entered with so much resolution upon this new course of life, that nothing since has been able to divert me from it. The consequence was, that in a few days I began to perceive that such a course agreed well with me; and, by pursuing it, I found myself in less than a year (some people, perhaps, will not believe it) entirely freed from all my complaints.

Having thus recovered my health, I began seriously to consider the power of temperance: if it had efficacy enough to subdue such grievous disorders as mine it must also have power to preserve me in health and strengthen my bad constitution. I therefore applied myself diligently to discover what kinds of food suited me best.

But, first, I resolved to try whether those which pleased my palate were agreeable to my stomach, so that I might judge of the truth of the proverb, which is so universally held, namely: —That, whatever pleases the palate, must agree with the stomach, or, that whatever is palatable must be wholesome and nourishing. The issue was, that I found it to be false, for I soon found that many things which pleased my palate, disagreed with my stomach. Having thus convinced myself that the proverb in question was false, I gave over the use of such meats and wincs as did not suit me, and chose those which by experience I found agreed well with me, taking only as much as I could easily digest, having strict regard to quantity as well as quality; and contrived matters so as never to cloy my stomach with eating or drinking, and always rose from the table with a disposition to eat and drink more. In this

I conformed to the proverb, which says, that a man to consult his health must check his appetite. Having in this manner conquered intemperance I betook myself entirely to a temperate and regular life, and this it was which effected me that alteration already mentioned, that is, in less than a year, it rid me of all those disorders which had taken such hold on me, and which appeared at the time incurable. It had likewise this other good effect, that I no longer experienced those annual fits of sickness, with which I used to be afflicted while I followed my ordinary free manner of eating and drinking. I also became exceedingly healthy, as I have continued from that time to this day; and for no other reason than that I never transgressed against regularity and strict moderation.

In consequence, therefore, of my taking such methods, I have always enjoyed, and, God be praised, still enjoy, the best of health. It is true, that, besides the two most important rules relative to eating and drinking, which I have ever been very scrupulous to observe (that is, not to take of either, more than my stomach could easily digest, and to use only those things which agree with me), I have carefully avoided, as far as possible, all extreme heat, cold, extraordinary fatigue, interruption of my usual hours of rest, and staying long in bad air. I likewise did all that lay in my power, to avoid those evils, which we do not find it so easy to remove: melancholy, hatred, and other violent passions, which appear to have the greatest influence on our bodies. I have not, however, been able to guard so well against these disorders, as not to suffer myself now and then to be hurried away by them. But I have discovered this fact, that these passions, have, in the main, no great influence over bodies governed by the two foregoing rules of eating and drinking. Galen, who was an eminent physician, has said, that, so long as he followed these two rules, he suffered but little from such disorders, so little, that they never gave him above a day's uneasiness. That what he says is true, I am a living witness, and so are many others who know me, and have seen me, how often I have been exposed to heats and colds, and disagreeable changes of weather, without taking harm, and have likewise seen me (owing to various misfortunes which have more than once befallen me) greatly disturbed in mind; these things, however, did me but little harm, whereas, other members of my family, who followed not my way of living, were greatly disturbed; such in a word, was their grief and dejection at seeing me involved in expensive law suits, commenced against me by great and powerful men, that, fearing I should be ruined, they were seized with great melancholy humor, with which intemperate bodies always abound, and such influence had it over their bodies, that they were carried off before their time; whereas, I suffered nothing on the occasion, as I had in me no superfluous humors of that kind; nay, in order to keep up my spirits, I brought myself to think that God had permitted these suits against me, in order to make me more sensible of my strength of body and mind; and that I should get the better of them with honor and advantage, as it, in fact, came to pass; for, at last, I obtained a decree exceedingly favorable to my fortune and character.

But I may go a step farther, and show how favorable to recovery is a temperate life, in case of accident. At the age of seventy years, I happened, as is often the case, to be in a coach, which, going at a smart rate, was upset, and in that condition drawn a considerable way before the horses could be stopped. I received so many shocks and bruises, that I was taken out with my head and body terribly battered, and a dislocated leg and arm. When the physicians saw me in so bad a plight, they concluded that in three days I should die, but thought they would try what bleeding and purging would do, in order to prevent inflammation and fever. But I, on the contrary, knowing that, by reason of the sober life I had lived for so many years, my blood was in good and pure condition, refused to be either purged or bled. I just caused my arm and leg to be set, and suffered myself to be rubbed with some oils, which they said were proper on the occasion. Thus, without using any other kind of remedy, I recovered, as I thought I should, without feeling the least alteration in myself, or any bad effects from the accident; a thing which appeared no less than miraculous in the eyes of the physicians. Hence, we may infer, that he who leads a sober and regular life, and commits no excess in his diet, can suffer but little from mental disorders or external accidents. On the contrary, I conclude, especially from the late trial I have had, that excesses in eating and drinking are often fatal. Four years ago, I consented to increase the quantity of my food by two ounces, my friends and relations having, for some time past, urged upon me the necessity of such increase, that the quantity I took was too little for one so advanced in years; against this, I urged that nature was content with little, and that with this small quantity I had preserved myself for many years in health and activity, that I believed as a man advanced in years, his stomach grew weaker, and therefore the tendency should be to lessen the amount of food rather than to increase. I further reminded them of the two proverbs, which say: he who has a mind to eat a great deal, must eat but little; eating little makes life long, and, living long, he must eat much; and the other proverb was: that, what we leave after making a hearty meal, does us more good than what we have eaten. But my arguments and proverbs were not able to prevent them teasing me upon the subject; therefore, not to appear obstinate, or affecting to know more than the physicians themselves, but above all, to please my family, I consented to the increase before mentioned; so that, whereas previous, what with bread, meat, the yolk of an egg, and soup, I ate as much as twelve ounces, neither more nor less, I now increased it to fourteen; and whereas before I drank but fourteen ounces of wine, I now increased it to sixteen. This increase, had, in eight days' time, such an effect upon me, that, from being cheerful and brisk, I began to be peevish and melancholy, so that nothing could please me. On the twelfth day, I was attacked with a violent pain in my side, which lasted twenty-two hours and was followed by a fever, which continued thirty-five days without any respite, insomuch that all looked upon me as a dead man; but, God be praised, I recovered, and I am positive that it was the great regularity I had observed for so many years, and that only, which rescued me from the jaws of death.

Orderly living is, doubtless, a most certain cause and foundation of health and long life; nay, I say it is the only true medicine, and whoever weighs the matter well, will come to this conclusion. Hence it is, that when the physician comes to visit a patient, the first thing he prescribes is regular living, and certainly to avoid excess. Now, if the patient after recovery should continue so to live, he could not be sick again, and if a very small quantity of food is sufficient to restore his health, then but a slight addition is necessary for the continuance of the same; and so, for the future, he would want neither physician nor physic. Nay, by attending to what I have said, he would become his own physician, and indeed, the best he could have, since, in fact, no man should be a perfect physician to any but himself. The reason is, that any man, by repeated trials, may acquire a perfect knowledge of his own constitution, the kinds of food and drink which agree with him best. These repeated trials are necessary, as there is a great variety in the nature and stomachs of persons. I found that old wine did not suit me, but that the new wines did; and, after long practice, I discovered that many things, which might not be injurious to others, were not good for me. Now, where is the physician who could have informed me which to take, and which to avoid, since I by long observation, could scarce discover these things.

It follows, therefore, that it is impossible to be a perfect physician to another. A man cannot have a better guide than himself, nor any physic better than a regular life. I do not, however, mean that for the knowledge and cure of such disorders as befall those who live an irregular life there is no occasion for a physician and that his assistance ought to be slighted; such persons should at once call in medical aid, in case of sickness. But, for the bare purpose of keeping ourselves in good health, I am of opinion, that we should consider this regular life as our physician, since it preserves men, even those of a weak constitution, in health; makes them live sound and hearty, to the age of one hundred and upward, and prevents their dying of sickness, or through the corruption of their humors, but merely by the natural decay, which at the last must come to all. These things, however, are discovered but by few, for men, for the most part, are sensual and intemperate, and love to satisfy their appetites, and to commit every excess; and, by way of apology, say that they prefer a short and self-indulgent life, to a long and self-denying one, not knowing that those men are most truly happy who keep their appetites in subjection. Thus have I found it, and I prefer to live temperately, so that I may live long and be useful. Had I not been temperate, I should never have written these tracts, which I have the pleasure of thinking will be serviceable to others. Sensual men affirm that no man can live a regular life. To this I answer, that Galen, who was a great physician, led such a life, and chose it as the best physic. The same did Plato, Cicero, Isocrates, and many other great men of former times, whom not to tire the reader I forbear naming; and, in our days, Pope Paul Farnese and Cardinal Bembo; and it was for that reason they lived so long. Therefore, since many have led this life, and many are actually leading it, surely all might conform to it, and the more so, as no great difficulty attends it. Cicero affirms that nothing is needed, but to be in good earnest. Plato, you say, though he himself lived thus regularly, affirms that, in republics, men often cannot do so, being obliged to expose themselves to various hardships and changes, which are incompatible with a regular life. I answer, that men who have to undergo these things, would be the better able to bear such hardships by being strictly temperate in matters of eating and drinking.

Here it may be objected, that he who leads this strict and regular life, having constantly when well made use only of simple food fit for the sick, and in small quantities, has when himself in sickness, no recourse left in matters of diet. To which I reply, that, whoever leads a regular life, cannot be sick or at least but seldom. By a regular life I mean, that a man shall ascertain for himself, how small a quantity of food and drink is sufficient to supply the daily wants of his nature and then having done this, and found out the kinds of food and drink best suited for his constitution, he shall, having formed his plans, strictly adhere to his resolutions and principles, not being careful at one time, and self-indulgent at others, for by so doing, he would gain but little benefit; but taking care always to avoid excess, which any man can certainly do at all times, and under all circumstances, if he is determined. I say then, that he who thus lives cannot be sick, or but seldom, and for a short time, because, by regular living, he destroys every seed of sickness, and thus, by removing the cause, prevents the effect; so that he who pursues a regular and strictly moderate life, need not fear illness, for his blood having become pure, and free from all bad humors, it is not possible that he can fall sick.

Since, therefore, it appears that a regular life is also profitable and virtuous, it ought to be universally followed, and more so, as it does not clash with duties of any kind, but is easy to all. Neither is it necessary that all should eat as little as I do—twelve ounces—or not to eat of many things from which I, because of the natural weakness of my stomach, abstain. Those with whom all kinds of food agree, may eat of such, only they are forbidden to eat a greater quantity, even of that which agrees with them best, than their stomachs can with ease digest. The same is to be understood of drink. The only rule for such to observe in eating and drinking, is the quantity rather than the quality; but for those who, like myself, are weak of constitution, these must not only be careful as to quantity, but also to quality, partaking only of such things as are simple, and easy to digest.

Let no one tell me that there are numbers, who, though they live most irregularly, attain in health and spirits to a great age. This argument is grounded on uncertainty and hazard, and such cases are rare. Men should not, therefore, because of these exceptional cases, be persuaded to irregularity or indulgence. Whoever, trusting to the strength of his constitution, slights these observations, may expect to suffer by so doing, and to live inconstant danger of disease and death. I therefore affirm, that a man, even of a bad constitution, who leads a strictly regular and sober life, is surer of a long one, than he of the best constitution who lives carelessly and irregularly. If men have a mind to live long and healthy, and die without sickness of body or mind, but by mere dissolution, they must submit to a regular and abstemious life, for such a life keeps the blood clean and pure. It suffers no vapors to ascend from the stomach to the head; hence, the brain of him who thus lives enjoys constant serenity; he can soar above the low and groveling concerns of this life to the exalted and beautiful contemplation of heavenly things to his exceeding comfort and satisfaction. He then truly discerns the brutality of those excesses into which men fall, and which bring them misery here and hereafter; while he may with comfort look forward to a long life, conscious that, through the mercy of God, he has relinquished the paths of vice and intemperance, never again to enter them; and, through the merits of our Saviour Jesus Christ, to die in His favor. He therefore does not suffer himself to be cast down with the thoughts of death, knowing that it will not attack him violently, or by surprise, or with sharp pains and feverish sensations, but will come upon him with ease and gentleness; like a lamp, the oil of which is exhausted, he will pass gently, and without any sickness, from this terrestrial and mortal, to a celestial and eternal life.

Some sensual unthinking persons affirm that a long life is no great blessing, and that the state of a man, who has passed his seventy-fifth year, cannot really be called life; but this is wrong, as I shall fully prove; and it is my sincere wish, that all men would endeavor to attain my age, that they might enjoy that period of life, which of all others is most desirable.

I will therefore give an account of my recreations, and the relish which I find at this stage of life. There are many who can give testimony as to the happiness of my life. In the first place, they see with astonishment the good state of my health and spirits; how I mount my horse without assistance, how I not only ascend a flight of stairs, but can climb a hill with greatest ease. Then, how gay and good-humored I am; my mind ever undisturbed, in fact, joy and peace having fixed there above in my breast. Moreover, they know in what manner I spend my time, so as never to find life weary: I pass my hours in great delight and pleasure, in converse with men of good sense and intellectual culture; then, when I cannot enjoy their company, I betake myself to the reading of some good book. When I have read as much as I like, I write; endeavoring in this, as in other things to be of service to others; and these things I do with the greatest ease to myself, living in a pleasant house in the most beautiful quarter of this noble city of Padua. Besides this house, I have my gardens, supplied with pleasant streams in which I always find something to do which amuses me. Nor are my recreations rendered less agreeable by the failing of any of my senses, for they are all, thank God, perfect, particularly my palate, which now relishes better the simple fare I have, than it formerly did the most delicate dishes, when I led an irregular life. Nor does the change of beds give me any uneasiness: I can sleep everywhere soundly and quietly, and my dreams are pleasant and delightful. It is likewise with the greatest pleasure I behold the success of an undertaking so important to this state; I mean that of draining and improving so many uncultivated pieces of ground, an undertaking begun within my memory, but which I thought I should never see completed; nevertheless I have, and was even in person assisting in the work for two months together, in those marshy places during the heat in summer, without ever finding myself worse for the fatigues or inconveniences I suffered; of so much efficacy is that orderly life, which I everywhere constantly lead. Such are some of the recreations and diversions of my old age, which is so much the more to be valued than the old age, or even the youth of other men; as, being freed by God's grace from the perturbations of the mind and the infirmities of the body, I no longer experience any of those contrary emotions which rack such a number of young men and as many old ones, who, by reason of their careless living and intemperate habits, are destitute of health and strength, and consequently of all true enjoyment.

And if it be lawful to compare little matters to affairs of importance, I will further venture to say that such are the effects of this sober life, that, at my present age of eighty-three, I have been able to write an entertaining comedy, abounding with innocent mirth and pleasant jests.

I have yet another comfort which I will mention; that of seeing a kind of immortality in a succession of descendants; for, as often as I return home, I find before me, not one or two, but eleven grandchildren, the oldest of them eighteen, all the offspring of one father and mother, and all blessed with good health. Some of the youngest I play with; those older, I make companions of; and, as nature has bestowed good voices upon them, I amuse myself by hearing them sing, and play on different instruments. Nay, I sing myself, as I have a better voice now, clearer and louder, than at any period of my life. Such are the recreations of my old age.

Whence it appears, that the life I lead is not gloomy, but cheerful, and I would not exchange my manner of living and my gray hairs, with that of even a young man, having the best constitution, who gave way to his appetites; knowing, as I do, that such are daily subject to a thousand kinds of ailments and death. I remember my own conduct in early life, and I know how foolhardy are young men; how apt they are to presume on their strength in all their actions, and by reason of their little experience, are over-sanguine in their expectations. Hence, they often expose themselves rashly to every kind of danger, and, banishing reason, bow their necks to the yoke of concupiscence, and endeavor to gratify all their appetites, not minding, fools as they are, that they thereby hasten the approach of what they would most willingly avoid, sickness and death.

And these are two great evils to all men who live a free life; the one is troublesome and painful, the other, dreadful and insupportable, especially when they reflect on the errors to which this mortal life is subject, and on the vengeance which the justice of God is wont to take on sinners. Whereas, I, in my old age, praise to the Almighty, am exempt from these torments; from the first, because I cannot fall sick, having removed all the cause of illness by my regularity and moderation; from the other, that of death, because from so many years' experience, I have learned to obey reason; whereas, I not only think it a great folly to fear that which cannot be avoided, but likewise firmly expect some consolation from the grace of Jesus Christ, when I arrive at that period.

But though I know I must, like others, reach that term, it is yet at so great a distance that I cannot discern it, because I know I shall not die except by mere dissolution, having already, by my regular course of life, shut up all other avenues of death, and thus prevented the humors of my body making any other way upon me, than that which I must expect from the elements employed in the composition of this mortal frame. I am not so simple as not to know that, as I was born, so I must die; but the natural death that I speak of does not overtake one, until after a long course of years; and even then, I do not expect the pain and agony which most men suffer when they die. But I, by God's blessing, reckon that I have still a long time to live in health and spirits, and enjoy this beautiful world, which is, indeed, beautiful to those who know how to make it so, but its beauty can only be realized by those who, by reason of temperance and virtue, enjoy sound health of body and mind.

Now, if this sober and moderate manner of living brings so much happiness; if the blessings that attend it are so stable and permanent, then I beseech every man of sound judgment to embrace this valuable treasure, that of a long and healthful life, a treasure which exceeds all other worldly blessings, and, therefore, should be sought after; for what is wealth and abundance to a man who is possessed with a feeble and sickly body? This is that divine sobriety, agreeable to God, the friend of nature, the daughter of reason, the sister of all the virtues, the companion of temperate living, modest, courteous, content with little, regular, and perfectly mistress of all her operations. From her, as from their proper root, spring life, health, cheerfulness, industry, learning and all those actions and employments worthy of noble and generous minds. The laws of God are all in her favor. Repletion, excess, intemperance, superfluous humors, diseases, fevers, pains and the dangers of death, vanish in her presence, as mists before the sun. Her comeliness ravishes every well-disposed mind. Her influence is so sure, as to promise to all a long and agreeable life. And, lastly, she promises to be a mild and pleasant guardian of life teaching how to ward off the attacks of death. Strict sobriety, in eating and drinking, renders the senses and understanding clear, the memory tenacious, the body lively and strong, the movements regular and easy; and the soul, feeling so little of her earthly burden, experiences much of her natural liberty. The man thus enjoys a pleasing and agreeable harmony, there being nothing in his system to disturb; for his blood is pure, and runs freely through his veins, and the heat of his body is mild and temperate.

The Second Discourse:

Showing the Surest Method of Correcting an Infirm Constitution

My treatise on a sober life has begun to answer my desire, in being of service to many persons born of a weak constitution, or who, by reason of free living, have become infirm, who, when they commit the least excess, find themselves greatly indisposed. I should also be glad to be of service to those, who, born with a good constitution, yet, by reason of a disorderly life, find themselves at the age of fifty or sixty attacked with various pains and diseases, such as gout, sciatica, liver and stomach complaints, to which they would not be subject, were they to live a strictly temperate life, and by so doing would moreover greatly increase the term of their existence, and live with much greater comfort; they would find themselves less irritable, and less disposed to be upset by inconvenience and annoyance. I was myself of a most irritable disposition, insomuch that at times there was no living with me. Now, for a very long time it has been otherwise, and I can see that a person swayed by his passions is little or no better than a madman at such times.

The man, also, who is of a bad constitution, may, by dint of reason, and a regular and sober life, live to a great age and in good health, as I have done, who had naturally one of the worst, so that it appeared impossible I should live above forty years, whereas, I now find myself sound and hearty at the age of eighty-six; forty-six years beyond the time I had expected; and during this long respite all my senses have continued perfect; and even my teeth, my voice, my memory, and my heart. But what is still more, my brain is clearer now than it ever was. Nor do any of my powers abate as I advance in life; and this because, as I grow older, I lessen the quantity of my solid food. This retrenchment is necessary, since it is impossible for man to live forever; and, as he draws near his end, he is brought so low as to be able to take but little nourishment, and at such times, the yolk of an egg, and a few spoonfuls of milk with bread, is quite sufficient during the twenty-four hours;

a greater quantity would most likely cause pain, and shorten life. In my own case, I expect to die without any pain or sickness, and this is a blessing of great importance; yet may be expected by those who shall lead a sober life, whether they be rich or poor. And, since a long and healthy life ought to be greatly coveted by every man, then I conclude that all men are in duty bound to exert themselves to that effect; nevertheless such a blessing cannot be obtained without strict temperance and sobriety. But some allege that many, without leading such a life, have lived to a hundred, and that in good health, though they ate a great deal, and used indiscriminately every kind of viands and wine, and therefore they flatter themselves that they shall be equally fortunate. But in this they are guilty of two mistakes: the first is, that it is not one in fifty thousand that ever attains that happiness; the other mistake is, that such, in the end, most certainly contract some illness, which carries them off: nor can they be sure of ending their days otherwise; so that the safest way to attain a long and healthful life, is to embrace sobriety, and to diet oneself strictly as to quantity. And this is no very difficult affair. History informs us of many who lived in the greatest temperance; and this present age furnishes us with many such, reckoning myself one of the number: we are all human beings, endowed with reason, and consequently we ought to be master of all our actions.

This sobriety is reduced to two things, quality and quantity. The first consists in avoiding food or drinks, which are found to disagree with the stomach. The second, to avoid taking more than the stomach can easily digest; and every man at the age of forty ought to be a perfect judge in these matters; and whoever observes these two rules, may be said to live a regular and sober life. And the virtue and efficacy of this life is such, that the humors in a man's blood become harmonious and perfect, and are no longer liable to be disturbed or corrupted by any disorders, such as suffering from excessive heat or cold, too much fatigue, or want of rest, and the like. A man who lives as I have described, may pass through all these changes without harm. Wherefore, since the humors of persons who observe these two rules relative to eating and drinking, cannot possibly be corrupted and engender acute diseases (the cause of untimely death), every man is bound to comply with them, for whoever acts otherwise, living a disorderly life, instead of a regular one, is constantly exposed to disease and death.

It is, indeed, true that even those who observe these two rules, relating to diet, the observance of which constitutes a regular life, may, by committing any one of the other irregularities, such as excessive heat, cold, fatigue, etc., find himself slightly indisposed for a day or two, but he need fear nothing worse.

But as there are some persons who, though well stricken in years, are, nevertheless, very free in their living, and allege that neither the quantity nor the quality of their diet makes any impression upon them, and therefore eat a great deal of everything without distinction, and indulge themselves equally in point of drinking; such men are ignorant of the requirements of their nature, or they are gluttonous; and I do affirm, that such do not enjoy good health, but as a rule are infirm, irritable, and full of maladies. There are others, who say that it is necessary that they should eat and drink freely to keep up their natural heat, which is constantly diminishing, as they advance in years; and that it is therefore their duty to eat heartily of such things as please their palate, and that strict moderation, in their case, would tend to shorten life. Now, this is the reason, or excuse, of thousands. But to all this, I answer, that all such are deceiving themselves, and I speak from experience, as well as observation. The fact is, large quantities of food cannot be digested by old stomachs; as man gets weaker as he grows older, and the waste in his system is slower, the natural heat certainly is less. Nor will all the food in the world increase it, except to bring on fever and distressing disorders; therefore, let none be afraid of shortening their days by eating too little. I am strong and hearty, and full of good spirits, neither have I ache or pain, and yet I am very old, and subsist upon very little; and, in this respect, that which would suit one man, is good for another. When men are taken ill they discontinue, or nearly so, their food. Now, if by reducing themselves to a small quantity, they recover from the jaws of death, how can they doubt, but that, with a slight increase of diet consistent with reason, they will be able to support nature, when in health. Let a fair, honest trial of some few weeks be given, and the result would, in all cases, be most pleasing.

Others say, that it is better for a man to suffer three or four times every year, from gout, sciatica, or whatever disorder to which he may be subject, than be tormented the whole year by not indulging his appetite, and eating and drinking just as he pleases, since he can always by a few days of self-denial recover from all such attacks. To this I answer, that, our natural heat growing less and less as we advance in years, no abstinence for a short time can have virtue sufficient to conquer the malady to which the man is subject, and which is generally brought on by repletion, so that he must die at last of one of these periodical disorders; for they abridge life in the same proportion as temperance and health prolong it.

Others pretend that it is better to live a short and self-indulgent life, than a long and self-denying one; but surely, longevity ought to be valued, and is, by men of good understanding; and those who do not truly prize this great gift of God, are surely a disgrace to mankind, and their death is a service to the public rather than not. And again, there are some, who, though they are conscious that they become weaker as they advance in years, yet cannot be brought to retrench the quantity of their food, but rather increase it, and, because they find themselves unable to digest the great quantity of food, with which they load their stomachs twice or thrice a day, they resolve to eat but once, heartily, in the twenty-four hours. But this course is useless; for the stomach is still overburdened, and the food is not digested, but turns into bad humors, by which the blood becomes poisoned, and thus a man kills himself long before his time. I never met with an aged person who enjoyed health, and lived that manner of life. Now, all these men whose manner of life I have named, would live long and happily, if, as they advanced in years, they lessened the quantity of their food, and ate oftener, and but little at a time, for old stomachs cannot digest large quantities; men at this age becoming children again, who eat little and often during the twenty-four hours.

O thrice holy sobriety, so useful to man, by reason of the service thou dost render him! Thou prolongest his days, by which means he greatly improves his understanding and, by such knowledge, he can avoid the bitter fruits of sensuality, which is an enemy to man's reason. Thou, moreover, freest him from the dreadful thoughts of death. How greatly ought we to be indebted to thee, since by thee we enjoy this beautiful world, which is really beautiful to all whose sensibilities have not been deadened by repletion, and whose minds have not been blighted by sensuality! I really never knew till I grew old, that the world was so beautiful; for, in my younger years I was debauched by irregularities, and therefore could not perceive and enjoy, as I do now, its beauties. O truly happy life, which, over and above all these favors conferred on me, hast so improved and perfected my body, that now I have a better relish for plain bread, than formerly I had for the most exquisite dainties! In fact I find such sweetness in it, because of the good appetite I always have, that I should be afraid of sinning against temperance, were I not convinced of the absolute necessity for it, and knowing that pure bread is, above all things, man's best food, and while he leads a sober life, he may be sure of never wanting that natural sauce, —a good appetite—and moreover, I find that, whereas I used to eat twice a day, now that I am much older, it is better for me to eat four times, and still to lessen the quantity as the years increase. And this is what I do, guided by my experience; therefore, my spirits being never oppressed by too much food, are always brisk; especially after eating, so that I enjoy much the singing of a song, before I sit down to my writing.

Nor do I ever find myself the worse for writing directly after meals; my understanding is never clearer; and I am never drowsy; the food I take being too small a quantity to send up any fumes to the brain. O, how advantageous it is to an old man to eat but little; therefore I take but just enough to keep body and soul together, and the things I eat are as follows: bread, panado, eggs (the yolk), and soups. Of flesh meat, I eat kid and mutton. I eat poultry of every kind; also of sea and river fish. Some men are too poor to allow themselves food of this kind, but they may do well on bread (made from wheat meal, which contains far more nutriment than bread made from fine flour), panado, eggs, milk, and vegetables. But though a man should eat nothing but these, he may not eat more than his stomach can with ease digest, never forgetting that it is the over-quantity which injures, even more than the eating of unsuitable food. And again I say, that whoever does not transgress, in point of either quantity or quality, cannot die, but by mere dissolution, except in cases where there is some inherited disease to combat; but such cases are comparatively rare, and even here a strict and sober diet will be of the greatest service.

O, what a difference between a regular and temperate life, and an irregular and intemperate life! One gives health and longevity, the other produces disease and untimely death. How many of my dearest relations and friends have I lost by their free living, whereas, had they listened to me, they might have been full of life and health. I am thus more than ever determined to use my utmost endeavors to make known the benefit of my kind of life. Here I am, an old man, yet full of life and joy, happier than at any previous period of my life, surrounded by many comforts; not the least to mention are my eleven grandchildren, all of fine understanding and amiable disposition, beautiful in their persons, and well disposed to learning; and these, I hope so to teach, that they shall take pattern after me, and follow my kind of life.

Now, I am often at a loss to understand why men of fine parts and understanding, who have attained middle age, do not, when they find themselves attacked by disorders and sickness, betake themselves to a regular life, and that constantly. Is it because they are in ignorance as to the importance of this subject? Surely, it cannot be that they are enslaved by their appetites to such an extent that they find themselves unable to adopt a strict and regular diet? As to young men, I am in no way surprised at their refusal to live such a life, for their passions are strong and usually their guide. Neither have they much experience; but, when a man has arrived at the age of forty of fifty, surely he should in all things be governed by reason. And this would teach men that gratifying the appetite and palate, is not, as many affirm, natural and right, but is the cause of disease and premature death. Were this pleasure of the palate lasting, it would be some excuse; but it is momentary, compared with the duration of the disease which its excess engenders. But it is a great comfort to a man of sober life to reflect, that what he eats will keep him in good health, and be productive of no disease or infirmity.

The Third Discourse:

The Method of Enjoying Complete Happiness in Old Age

My Lord,

In writing to your Lordship, it is true I shall speak of few things, but such as I have already mentioned in my essays, but I am sure your Lordship will not tire of the repetition.

My Lord, to begin, I must tell you, that being now at the age of ninety-one, I am more sound and hearty than ever, much to the amazement of those who know me. I, who can account for it, am bound to show that a man can enjoy a terrestrial paradise after eighty; but it is not to be obtained, except by strict temperance in food and drink, virtues acceptable to God and friends to reason. I must, however, go on to tell you, that, during the past few days I have been visited by many of the learned doctors of this university, as well as physicians and philosophers who were well acquainted with my age, life, and manners, also, that I was stout, hearty, and lively, my senses perfect, also my voice and teeth, likewise my memory and judgment. They knew, besides, that I constantly employed eight hours every day in writing treatises, with my own hand, on subjects useful to mankind, and spent many more in walking and singing. O, my Lord, how melodious my voice is grown! Were you to hear me chant my prayers, and that to my lyre, after the example of David, I am certain it would give you great pleasure, my voice is so musical.

Now, these doctors and philosophers told me that it was next to a miracle, that at my age, I should be able to write upon subjects which required both judgment and spirit, and added that I ought not to be looked upon as a person advanced in years, since all my occupations were those of a young man, and that I was altogether unlike aged people of seventy and eighty, who are subject to various ailments and diseases, which render life a weariness; or, if even any by chance escape these things, yet their senses are impaired, sight, or hearing, or memory is defective, and all their faculties much decayed; they are not strong, nor cheerful, as I am. And they moreover said, that they looked upon me as having special grace conferred upon me, and said a great many eloquent and fine things, in endeavoring to prove this, which, however, they could not do; for their arguments were not grounded on good and sufficient reasons, but merely on their opinions. I therefore endeavored to undeceive and set them right, and convince them that the happiness I enjoyed was not confined to me, but might be common to all mankind, since I was but a mere mortal, and different in no respect from other men, save in this, that I was born more weakly than some, and had not what is called a strong constitution. Man, however, in his youthful days, is more prone to be led by sensuality than reason; yet, when he arrives at the age of forty, or earlier, he should remember that he has about reached the summit of the hill, and must now think of going down, carrying the weight of years with him; and that old age is the reverse of youth, as much as order is the reverse of disorder; hence, it is requisite that he should alter his mode of life in regard to the quality and quantity of his food and drink. For it is impossible in the nature of things, that the man who is bent on indulging his appetite, should be healthy and free from ailments. Hence it was to avoid this vice and its evil effects, I embraced a regular and sober life. It is no doubt true, that I at first found some difficulty in accomplishing this, but in order to conquer the difficulty I besought the Almighty to grant the virtue of sobriety in all things, well knowing that He would graciously hear my prayer. Then, considering that when a man is about to undertake a thing of importance, which he knows he can compass, though not without difficulty, he may make it much easier to himself by being steady in his purpose, I pursued this course: I endeavored gradually to relinquish a disorderly life, and to suit myself to strict temperate rules; and this it came to pass, that a sober and moderate life no longer became disagreeable, though, on account of the weakness of my constitution, I tied myself down to very strict rules in regard to the quantity and quality of what I ate and drank.

Others, who happen to be blessed with a strong constitution, may eat a greater variety of food, and in somewhat larger quantity, each man being a guide to himself, consulting always his judgment and reason, rather than his fancy or appetite, and further let him always strictly abide by his rules, for he will receive little benefit if he occasionally indulges in excess.

Now, on hearing these arguments, and examining the reasons on which they were founded, the doctors and philosophers agreed that I had advanced nothing but what was true. One of the younger of them said that I appeared to enjoy the special grace of being able to relinquish, with ease, one kind of life, and embrace another, a thing which he knew from theory to be feasible, but in practice to be difficult, for it had proved as hard to him, as easy to me.

To this I replied, that, being human like himself, I likewise had found it no easy task, but it did not become a man to shrink from a glorious and practical task, on account of its difficulties; the greater the obstacles to overcome, the greater the honor and benefit. Our beneficent Creator is desirous, that, as He originally favored human nature with longevity, we should all enjoy the full advantage of His intentions, knowing that when a man has passed seventy, he may be exempt from the sensual strivings, and govern himself entirely by the dictates of reason. Vice and immorality then leave him, and God is willing that he should live to the full maturity of his years, and has ordained that all who reach their natural term should end their days without sickness, but by mere dissolution, the natural way; the wheels of life quietly stopping, and man peacefully leaving this world, to enter upon immortality, as will be my case; for I am sure to die thus, perhaps while chanting my prayers. Nor do the thoughts of death give me the least concern; nor does any other thought connected with death, namely, the fear of the punishment to which wicked men are liable, because I am bound to believe, that being a Christian, I shall be saved by the virtue of the most sacred blood of Jesus Christ, which He freely shed in order to save those who trust in Him. Thus, how beautiful my life! How happy my end! To this, the young doctor had nothing to reply, but that he would follow my example.

The great desire I had, my Lord, to converse with you at this distance, has forced me to be prolix, and still obliges me to proceed, though not much farther. There are some sensualists, my

Lord, who say that I have thrown away my time and trouble, in writing a treatise upon temperance, and other discourses on the same subject; alleging, that it is impossible to conform to it, so that my treatise must answer as little purpose as that of Plato on Government, who took a great deal of pains to recommend a thing impracticable. Now, this much surprises me, as they may see that I lived a sober life many years before I wrote my treatise, and I should never have composed it, had I not been convinced, that it was such a life as any man might lead; and being a virtuous life, would be of great service to him; so that I felt myself under an obligation to present it in its true light. Again, I have the satisfaction to hear that numbers, on reading my treatise, have embraced such a life. So that the objection concerning Plato on Government is of no force against my case. But a sensualist is an enemy to reason, and a slave to his passions.

The Fourth Discourse:

An Exhortation to a Sober and Regular Life in Order to Attain Old Age

Not to be wanting in my duty, and not to lose at the same time the satisfaction I feel in being useful to others, I again take up my pen to inform those, who, for want of conversing with me, are strangers to what those with whom I am acquainted, know and see. But as some things may appear to certain persons scarcely credible, though actually true, I shall not fail to relate for the benefit of the public. Wherefore, I say, being arrived at my ninety-fifth year, God be praised, and still finding myself sound and hearty, content and cheerful, I never cease to thank the Divine Majesty for so great a blessing, considering the usual condition of old men. These scarcely ever attain the age of seventy, without losing health and spirits, and growing melancholy and peevish. Moreover, when I remember how weak and sickly I was between the ages of thirty and forty, and how from the first, I never had what is called a strong constitution; I say, when I remember these things, I have surely abundant cause for gratitude, and though I know I cannot live many years longer, the thought of death gives me no uneasiness; I, moreover, firmly believe that I shall attain to the age of one hundred years. But, to render this dissertation more methodical, I shall begin by considering man at his birth; and from thence accompany him through every stage of life, to his grave.

I therefore say, that some come into the world with the stamina of life so weak, that they live but a few days, or months, or years, and it is not always easy to show, to what the shortness of life is owing. Others are born sound and lively, but still, with a poor, weakly constitution; and of these, some live to the age of ten, twenty, others to thirty or forty, but seldom live to be old men. Others, again, bring into the world a perfect constitution, and live to an old age; but it is generally, as I have said, an old age of sickness and sorrow, for which usually they have to thank themselves, because they unreasonably presumed on the goodness of their constitution; and cannot by any means be brought to alter when grown old, from the mode of life they pursued in their younger days, but live as irregularly when past the meridian of life, as they did in the time of their youth. They do not consider that the stomach has lost much of its natural heat and vigor, and that, therefore, they should pay great attention to the quality and quantity of what they eat and drink; but, rather than decrease, many of them are for increasing the quantity, saying, that, as health and vigor grow less, they should endeavor to repair the loss by a great abundance of food, since it is by sustenance we are to preserve ourselves.

But it is here that the great mistake is made; since, as the natural force and heat lessen as a man grows in years, he should diminish the quantity of his food and drink, as nature at that period is content with little; and moreover, if increasing the amount of nourishment was the proper thing, then, surely the majority of men would live to a great age in the best of health. But do we see it so? On the contrary, such a case is a rare exception; whilst my course of life is proved to be right, by reason of its results. But, though some have every reason to believe this to be the case, they nevertheless, because of their lack of strength of character, and their love of repletion, still continue their usual manner of living. But were they, in due time, to form strict temperate habits, they would not grow infirm in their old age, but would continue as I am, strong and hearty, and might live to the age of one hundred, or one hundred and twenty. This has been the case with others of whom we read, men who were born with a good constitution, and lived sober and abstemious lives; and had it been my lot to have enjoyed a strong constitution, I should make no doubt of attaining to that age. But as I was born feeble, and with an infirm constitution, I am afraid I shall not outlive an hundred years; and were others, born weakly as myself, to betake them to a life like mine, they would, like me, live to the age of a hundred, as shall be my case.

And this certainty of being able to live to a great age is, in my opinion, a great advantage (of course I do not include accidents, to which all are liable, and which must specially be left to our Maker), and highly to be valued; none being sure of this blessing, except such as adhere to the rules of temperance. This security of life is built on good and truly natural reasons, which can never fail; it being impossible that he who leads a perfectly sober and temperate life, should breed any sickness, or die before his time. Sooner, he cannot through ill-health die, as his sober life has the virtue to remove the cause of sickness, and sickness cannot happen without a cause; which cause being removed, sickness is also removed, and untimely and painful death prevented.

And there is no doubt, that temperance in food and drink, taking only as much as nature really requires, and thus being guided by reason, instead of appetite, has efficacy to remove all cause of disease; for since health and sickness, life and death, depend on the good or bad condition of a man's blood, and the quality of his humors, such a life as I speak of purifies the blood, and corrects all vicious humors, rendering all perfect and harmonious. It is true, and cannot be denied, that man must at last die, however careful with himself he may have been; but yet, I maintain, without sickness and great pain; for in my case I expect to pass away quietly and peacefully, and my present condition insures this to me, for, though at this great age, I am hearty and content, eating with a good appetite, and sleeping soundly. Moreover, all my senses are as good as ever, and in the highest perfection; my understanding clear and bright, my judgment sound, my memory tenacious, my spirits good, and my voice (one of the first things which is apt to fail us) has grown so strong and sonorous, that I cannot help chanting aloud my prayers, morning and night, instead of whispering and muttering them to myself as was formerly my custom.

O, how glorious is this life of mine, replete with all the felicities which man can enjoy on this side of the grave! It is entirely exempt from that sensual brutality, which age has enabled my reason to banish; thus I am not troubled with passions, and my mind is calm, and free from all perturbations, and doubtful apprehensions. Nor can the thought of death find room in my mind, at least, not in any way to disturb me. And all this has been brought about, by God's mercy, through my careful habit of living. How different from the life of most old men, full of aches and pains, and forebodings, whilst mine is a life of real pleasure, and I seem to spend my days in a perpetual round of amusements, as I shall presently show.

And first, I am of service to my country, and what a joy is this. I find infinite delight in being engaged in various improvements, in connection with the important estuary or harbor of this city, and fortifications; and although this Venice, this Queen of the Sea, is very beautiful, yet I have devised means by which it may be made still more beautiful, and more wealthy, for I have shown in what way she may abound with provisions, by improving large tracts of land, and bringing marshes and barren sand under cultivation. Then again, I have another great joy always present before me. Some time since, I lost a great part of my income, by which my grandchildren would be great losers. But I, by mere force of thought, have found a true and infallible method of repairing such loss more than double, by a judicious use of that most commendable of arts, agriculture. Another great comfort to me is to think that my treatise on temperance is really useful, as many assure me by word of mouth, and others by letter, where they say, that, under God they are indebted to me for their life. I have also much joy in being able to write, and am thus of service to myself and others; and the satisfaction I have in conversing with men of ability and superior understanding is very great, from whom I learn something fresh. Now, what a comfort is this, that old as I am, I am able, without fatigue of mind or body thus to be fully engaged, and to study the most important, difficult, and sublime subjects.

I must further add, that at this age, I appear to enjoy two lives: one terrestrial, which in fact I possess, the other celestial, which I possess in thought; and this thought is actual enjoyment, when founded upon things we are sure to attain, and I, through the infinite mercy and goodness of God, am sure of eternal life. Thus, I enjoy the terrestrial life in consequence of my sobriety and temperance, virtues so agreeable to the Deity, and I enjoy, by the grace of God, the celestial, which He makes me anticipate in thought; a thought so lively, as to fix me entirely on this subject, the fruition of which I hold to be of the utmost certainty. And I further maintain, that, dying in the manner I expect, is not really death, but a passage of the soul from this earthly life to a celestial, immortal, and infinitely perfect existence. Neither can it be otherwise; and this thought is so pleasing, so superlatively sublime, that it can no longer stoop to low and worldly objects, such as the death of this body, being entirely taken up with the happiness of living a celestial and divine life. Whence it is, that I enjoy two lives; and the thought of terminating this earthly life gives me no concern, for I know that I have a glorious and immortal life before me.

Now, is it possible, that any one should grow tired of so great a comfort and blessing as this which I enjoy, and which the majority of persons might attain, by leading the life I have led, an example which every one has it in his power to follow? For I am no saint, but a mere man, a servant of God, to whom so regular a life is extremely agreeable.

Now, there are men who embrace a spiritual and contemplative life, and this is holy and commendable, their chief employment being to celebrate the praises of God, and to teach men how to serve Him. Now, if while these men set themselves apart for this life, they would also betake themselves to sober and temperate living, how much more agreeable would they render themselves in the sight of God and men. What a much greater honor and ornament would they be to the world. They would likewise enjoy constant health and happiness, would attain a great age, and thus become eminently wise and useful; whereas, now, they are mostly infirm, irritable, and dissatisfied, and think that their various trials and ailments are sent them by Almighty God, with a view of promoting their salvation; that they may do penance in this life for their past errors. Now, I cannot help saying, that in my opinion, they are greatly mistaken; for I cannot believe that the Deity desires that man, his favorite creature, should be infirm and melancholy, but rather, that he should enjoy good health and be happy. Man, however, brings sickness and disease upon himself, by reason, either of his ignorance or willful self-indulgence. Now, if those who profess to be our teachers in divine matters would also set the example, and thus teach men how to preserve their bodies in health, they would do much to make the road to heaven easier: men need to be taught that self-denial and strict temperance is the path to health of body and health of mind, and those who thus live see more clearly than others what their duty is toward our Saviour

Jesus Christ, who came down upon earth to shed His precious blood, in order to deliver us from the tyranny of the devil, such was His immense goodness and loving kindness to man.

Now, to make an end of this discourse, I say, that since length of days abounds with so many favors and blessings, and I, not by theory, but by blessed experience can testify to it–indeed, I solemnly assure all mankind that I really enjoy a great deal more than I can mention, and that I have no other reason for writing, but that of demonstrating the great advantages, which arise from longevity, and such a life as I have lived—I desire to convince men, that they may be induced to observe these excellent rules of constant temperance in eating and drinking, and therefore, I never cease to raise my voice, crying out to you, my friends, that your lives may be even as mine.

Printed in Great Britain
by Amazon

36433497R00021